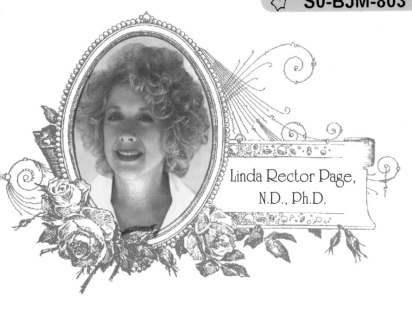

Linda Rector Page,
N.D., Ph.D.

Renewing Female Balance

P.M.S.
Breast & Uterine Fibroids
Ovarian Cysts
Endometriosis
Yeast Infections
&
More

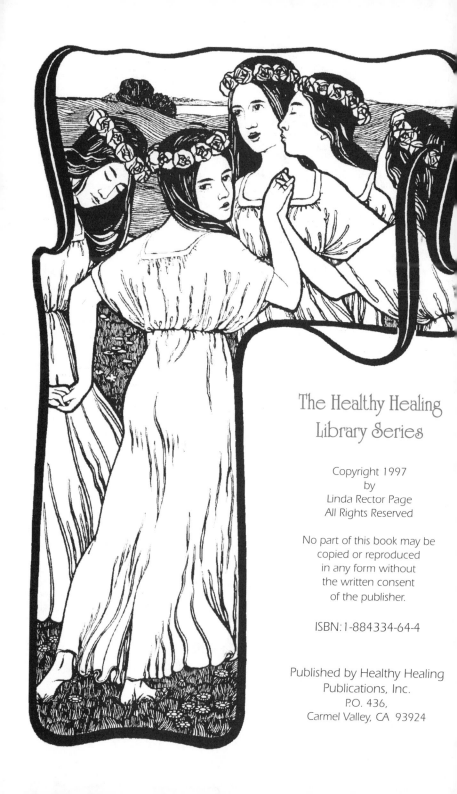

The Healthy Healing
Library Series

Copyright 1997
by
Linda Rector Page
All Rights Reserved

No part of this book may be
copied or reproduced
in any form without
the written consent
of the publisher.

ISBN: 1-884334-64-4

Published by Healthy Healing
Publications, Inc.
P.O. 436,
Carmel Valley, CA 93924

About the Author....

L inda Rector Page has been working in the fields of nutrition and herbal medicine both professionally and as a personal lifestyle choice, since the early seventies. She is a certified Doctor of Naturopathy and Ph.D., with extensive experience in formulating and testing herbal combinations. She received a Doctorate of Naturopathy from the Clayton School of Holistic Healing in 1988, and a Ph.D. in Nutritional Therapy from the American Holistic College of Nutrition in 1989. She is a member of both the American and California Naturopathic Medical Associations.

Linda opened and operated the "Rainbow Kitchen," a natural foods restaurant, then became a working partner in The Country Store Natural Foods store. She has written four successful books and a Library Series of specialty books in the nutritional healing field. Today, she lectures around the country and in the media on a wide range of natural healing topics.

Linda is the founder and formulator of Crystal Star Herbal Nutrition, a manufacturer of over 250 premier herbal compounds. A major, cutting edge influence in the herbal medicine field, Crystal Star Herbal Nutrition products are carried by over twenty-five hundred natural food stores in the U.S. and around the world.

Continuous research in all aspects of the alternative healing world has been the cornerstone of success for her reference work Healthy Healing now in its tenth edition. Feedback from all these sources provides up-to-the-minute contact with the needs, desires and results being encountered by people taking more responsibility for their own health. Much of the lifestyle information and empirical observation detailed in her books comes from this direct experience.

Cooking For Healthy Healing, now in its second revised edition, is a companion to Healthy Healing. It draws on both the recipes from the Rainbow Kitchen and the more defined, lifestyle diets that she has developed for healing since then. The book contains thirty-three diet programs, and over 900 healthy recipes.

In How To be Your Own Herbal Pharmacist, Linda addresses the rising appeal of herbs and herbal healing in America. This book is designed for those wishing to take more definitive responsibility for their health through individually developed herbal combinations.

Linda's newest work is a party reference book called Party Lights, written with restaurateur and chef Doug Vanderberg. Party Lights, takes healthy cooking one step further by adding in the fun to a good diet.

Published by Healthy Healing Publications, 1997

Bibliography & Other Reading

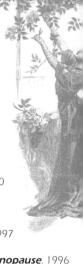

Gladstar, Rosemary. **Herbal Healing For Women**. 1993

Lark, Susan M., M.D. **Fibroid Tumors & Endometriosis**. 1995

Lark, Susan M., M.D. **Woman's Health Companion**. 1995

Stein, Diane. **The Natural Remedy Book for Women**. 1995

Lee, John R., M.D. **Natural Progesterone**. 1993

Hobbs, Christopher. **Vitex:The Woman's Herb**. Botanica Press, 1990

Santillo, Humbart, B.S., **M.H. Natural Healing with Herbs**. 1991

Light, Luise. "Kitchen Medicine for Women." *Vegetarian Times*. July 1997

Lee, John R., M.D. **What Your Doctor May Not Tell You About Menopause**. 1996

Hurley, Judith Benn. "A Women's Medicine Chest". *Vegetarian Times*. July 1996

Weiner, Michael, M.S., M.A. Ph.D. "Herbs for Women", *Herbal Healthline*. 1991

Whitaker, Dr. Julian. **Guide To Natural Healing**. Rocklin: Prima Publications, 1994.

Weiner, Michael A., M.S., M.A., Ph.D. "Herbs for Women: Part 1", *Herbal Healthline*.

Wright, Jonathan V., M.D. "Fibrocystic Breasts", *Nutrition & Healing*. July 1995.

Gaby, Alan R., M.D., *On PMS, Nutrition & Healing*. Vol. 1, Issue 3. Oct. 1994.
Gaby, Alan R., M.D., "Commentary" (on Fibro. Breasts), *Nutrition & Healing*. 1995.

Boyle, C.A., Berkowitz, G.S., LiVolsi, V.A., et al. "Caffeine Consumption and Fibrocystic Breast Disease: A Case-Control Epidemiologic Study", JNCI, 1984; 72: 1015-19.

Murray, Michael, N.D. and Joseph Pizzorno, M.D. **Encyclopedia of Natural Medicine.** Rocklin: Prima Publications, 1994.

Wright, Jonathan V., M.D. "Premenstrual Syndrome", *Nutrition & Healing*. Vol. 1, Issue 3. Oct. 1994.

Duke, J.A. **Handbook of Medicinal Herbs**. CRC Press, Boca Raton, FL 1985.

Hudson, Tori, N.D. "Fibrocystic Breast Disease...Or Is It?" Townsend Letter for Doctors. May 1994.

Donsbach, Kurt W., D.C., N.D., Ph.D. **PMS & Menopause & Hysterectomy.** The Rockland Corp., 1993.

Journal
Books
In

The Library Series

※   Renewing Female Balance
※   Do You Have Blood Sugar Blues?
※   A Fighting Chance For Weight Loss & Cellulite Control
※   The Energy Crunch & You
※   Gland & Organ Health - Taking Deep Body Care
※   Heart & Circulation - Controlling Blood Cholesterol
※   Detoxification & Body Cleansing to Fight Disease
※   Allergy Control & Management; Fighting Asthma
※   Ageless Vitality - Revealing the Secrets of Anti-Aging
※   Stress Management, Depression & Addictions
※   Colds & Flu & You - Building Optimum Immunity
※   Fighting Infections with Herbs - Controlling STDs
※   Beautiful Skin, Hair & Nails Naturally
※   Don't Let Your Food Go to Waste - Better Digestion
※   Do You Want to Have a Baby? Natural Prenatal Care
※   Menopause & Osteoporosis: - Taking Charge
※   Boosting Immunity With Power Plants
※   Herbal Therapy For Kids
※   Renewing Male Health & Energy
※   Cancer - Can Alternative Therapies Really Help?
※   Fatigue Syndromes - CFS, Candida, Lupus, Fibromyalgia & More
※   Overcoming Arthritis With Natural Therapies

Dr. Page's written papers are thoroughly researched - through empirical observation as well as from documented evidence. Studies are ongoing and updated at Healthy Healing Publications, P.O. Box 436, Carmel Valley, CA 93924.

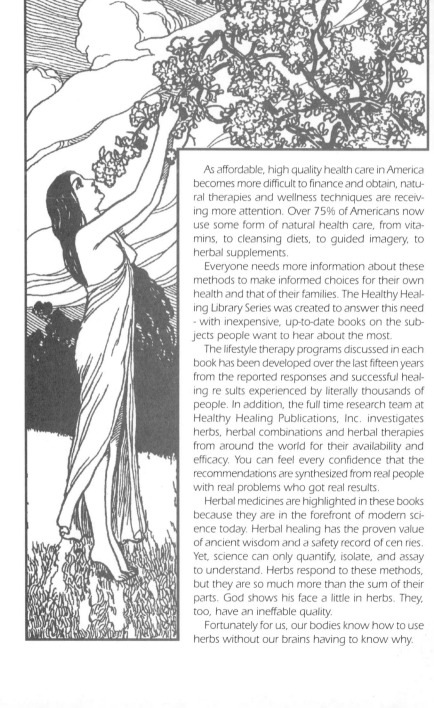

As affordable, high quality health care in America becomes more difficult to finance and obtain, natural therapies and wellness techniques are receiving more attention. Over 75% of Americans now use some form of natural health care, from vitamins, to cleansing diets, to guided imagery, to herbal supplements.

Everyone needs more information about these methods to make informed choices for their own health and that of their families. The Healthy Healing Library Series was created to answer this need - with inexpensive, up-to-date books on the subjects people want to hear about the most.

The lifestyle therapy programs discussed in each book has been developed over the last fifteen years from the reported responses and successful healing re sults experienced by literally thousands of people. In addition, the full time research team at Healthy Healing Publications, Inc. investigates herbs, herbal combinations and herbal therapies from around the world for their availability and efficacy. You can feel every confidence that the recommendations are synthesized from real people with real problems who got real results.

Herbal medicines are highlighted in these books because they are in the forefront of modern science today. Herbal healing has the proven value of ancient wisdom and a safety record of cen ries. Yet, science can only quantify, isolate, and assay to understand. Herbs respond to these methods, but they are so much more than the sum of their parts. God shows his face a little in herbs. They, too, have an ineffable quality.

Fortunately for us, our bodies know how to use herbs without our brains having to know why.

Table of Contents

Renewing Female Balance & Energy   Pg. 8
    The Wonders of the Female System   pg. 8
    Lifestyle Factors for Women's Health   pg. 9

Pre-Menstrual Syndrome - a New Epidemic?   Pg. 9
    A PMS Diet   pg. 11
    Herbal Therapy to Rebalance   pg. 13
    Addressing Specific PMS Problems   pg. 16

Endometriosis & Natural Therapies   Pg. 22
    Diet Therapy is Important   pg. 23
    A Successful Herbal Program   pg. 25
    About Wild Yam Creams   pg. 27

Natural Therapies Reduce Fibroids   Pg. 28
    A 3-Point Prevention Program   pg. 32
    Eliminating & Reducing Fibroids   pg. 33

Ovarian Cysts - You May Not Need Surgery   Pg. 36
    A Diet to Improve Body Chemistry   pg. 37
    Herbal Hormone Balancers   pg. 38

Relief For Vaginal Yeast Infections   Pg. 39
    Antibiotics/Probiotics & Yeasts   pg. 40
    Effective Natural Therapies   pg. 41

Sexually Transmitted Diseases & Women   Pg. 43
    Natural Therapy Offers a Choice   pg. 44

Renewing Female Balance & Energy

The female system is an incredibly beautiful, complex balance. It is an individual model of the creative universe.

A woman is usually a marvelous thing to be, but the intricacies of her body are delicately tuned and can become unbalanced or obstructed easily, causing pain, and poor function. A woman is such a wholly bound-together person that imbalances often cause lack of union between mind and body. She loses the accustomed oneness with herself, resulting in physiological and emotional problems.

> *From time immemorial women have been close to the Earth as part of the creative process. Herbs, important nutrients of the Earth's regenerating design, are primarily body balancers - and so work amazingly well with a woman's system.*

Drugs, chemicals and synthetic medicines stand outside this natural cycle, and often do not bring positive results for women. These substances usually try to add something to her body, or act symptomatically on a problem area. Yet, many female problems are caused by **overstimulation** of the glands by synthetically reproduced substances.

In fact, most of the serious disease women face today, like candida overgrowth, vaginal and urinary tract infections, auto-immune and sexually transmitted diseases, even cancer have been linked to modern synthetic chemicals and toxic environmental pollutants – and to the low nutritional value of America's mass processed foods.

I see it every day - women's natural feel for the Earth and their environment as critical to our culture's renewed knowledge of preventive health care. Women are leading the way by consciously creating programs for overall good health, with their own individual needs in mind.

A good diet is of utmost importance for a woman. A good diet maintains harmonious system balance, provides a high level of energy, keeps memory and thinking sharp, staves off disease, and contributes to a more youthful appearance. A diet of fresh, whole foods and juices, high fiber, low fats, cultured foods and plenty of pure water is imperative to her long term health. Concentrated proteins like animal foods, milk products, caffeine-containing foods, and sugary foods are best eaten in moderate amounts.

Regular exercise is pivotal to a woman's health, because it is a readily available antioxidant that enhances her immunity, raises calorie burning metabolism, boosts circulation, strengthens her bones and helps her deal with unhealthy emotion and stress.

Herbs are significant healing agents for women. *Women can have a great deal of confidence that herbal therapy will work for them. Herbs are in the forefront of modern science today with the proven value of ancient wisdom that women prize.*

Herbs are foundation body balancers, working through the glands, nourishing the body's most basic elements. Results will seem to take much longer than the quick effects of drugs. But this fact shows how herbs actually work - as support to control and reverse the cause of a problem, with more permanent effect.

Herbs work with a woman's own hormone action. As foods, herbs are identified and used by the body's own enzyme action. A woman's delicate system responds to them easily and safely. They are broad-based, gentle but effective nutrients that encourage the body to do its own work and to restore its own balance. Relief is often quite gratifying because it signifies healing within the body versus the suppression of symptoms. Most herbs, as edible plant foods, are as safe to take as foods.

I find that most women know their own bodies better than anyone else. They intuitively pinpoint their body systems that need rebalance, and often instinctively choose the herbal combination that will work best for them.

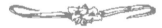

Women & Premenstrual Syndrome

Forget your period.....PMS is the real curse! Almost every woman we know has PMS in some form or other. It is by far the most common of all women's health complaints. There are new clinical estimations that a whopping 90% of all women between the ages of 20 and 50 experience PMS in varying degrees.

PMS symptoms tend to get worse for women in their late thirties and beyond. They are often magnified after taking birth control pills, after pregnancy and just before menopause because of hormone imbalances. We especially hate PMS because we feel out of control of our bodies. For some women, it disrupts their whole lives.

Premenstrual syndrome covers a wide variety of symptoms. Over 150 have been documented, and new ones are being added every year.

The most common symptoms include fatigue, swollen, tender breasts, abdominal bloating, swelling of hands and feet, depression, headaches, irritability, increased appetite, (especially cravings for sweet and salty foods), facial blemishes, insomnia, constipation and unusual emotional displays.

PMS symptoms have even been subdivided into groups: Type A (for anxiety), is characterized by irritability, anxiety, and mood swings. Eighty percent of women with PMS fall into this group. Type C (for cravings), is associated with cravings, increased appetite, lack of energy and headaches. Sixty percent of women with PMS have these symptoms. Type H (for hyperhydration or bloating), involves abdominal bloating and fluid retention in the hands feet and ankles, breast tenderness, and weight gain greater than three pounds. About fifty percent of women report these symptoms; and Type D (for depression), includes crying, confusion, forgetfulness, insomnia and sometimes serious depression. About twenty percent of women experience these feelings before their periods. Most women experience symptoms from more than one group.

The hormone shift in estrogen-to-progesterone ratios that women experience during the menstrual cycle appears to be the major factor in PMS symptoms. Most women have the widest variety of symptoms in the two week period before menstruation, when the estrogen/progesterone ratios are the most elevated.

Why wasn't PMS a big deal for our mothers and grandmothers? Is something different going on with women's bodies today?

PMS seems to be partially a consequence of the modern woman's emancipation. In times past, women were a silent, long-suffering lot, who felt the symptoms were just part of being a woman. Women were not out in the high profile workplace with men, and they could go to bed and suffer alone. In addition, our diets in times past consisted of more whole and fresh foods than they do today. The environment wasn't full of chemicals nor our foods full of junk.

With such a broad spectrum of symptoms affecting every system of the body, there is clearly no one treatment. Indeed the medical establishment has not been successful in addressing PMS with drugs. Natural therapies and a holistic approach show far more beneficial results, because self care allows a woman to tailor treatment to her own needs.

A woman can expect a natural therapy program for PMS to take at least two months as the body works through both ovary cycles with nutritional support. The first month, there is noticeable decrease in PMS symptoms; the second month finds them dramatically reduced. However, PMS is complex. Numerous body functions are tied into hormone secretions and gland cycles. Don't be discouraged if you need 6 months to gently coax your system into balance. Continuing with a good diet, and lower doses of your herb and/or vitamin choices, makes sense toward preventing PMS return even after most of the symptoms are gone.

What are the lifestyle keys to controlling PMS?

Lifestyle therapy, including a highly nutritious diet, herbal compounds, and food-derived vitamins, allows absorption through your body's own enzyme action. These nutrients encourage the body to do its own work, providing more permanent balance and relief.

≫Diet directly affects PMS. Improve your diet first to prevent it. A low fat, vegetarian diet with some fish and seafood produces good results in terms of diminished symptoms. Women with severe PMS symptoms consume 60% more refined carbohydrates, 280% more refined sugars, 85% more dairy products, and 80% more sodium than women who don't get PMS.

≫Reduce your dairy product consumption. Many dairy foods are also a source of synthetic estrogen from hormones injected into cows. Switch to nonfat dairy products. Estrogen is stored in fat, and non-fat foods don't contribute to estrogen stores. Nonfat yogurt is a good choice because it also contains digestive lactobacillus. On PMS days, dairy products should be avoided altogether because they are so congestive.

≫Cut back on sugar before your period. Sugar depletes the body's B-complex vitamins, increases sodium retention, and worsens the blood sugar problems many women experience before menses. Sugar also decreases magnesium by increasing its excretion in the urine.

≫Go low-salt for less PMS... especially before menses, to decrease fluid retention. (Extra potassium intake helps counterbalance salt's effects.)

≫A little wine is fine, but hard liquor should be avoided to control PMS. Alcohol lowers vitamin B levels and compromises liver function, reducing the liver's ability to break down excess estrogen.

⇒ **Reduce caffeine to one cup of coffee or less a day.** Several studies show a link between the amount of caffeine consumed and the severity of PMS. Caffeine depletes the body's store of B vitamins and contributes to anxiety, mood swings, and irritability. Fifteen to 30 percent of women with breast tenderness find relief by stopping caffeine use.

⇒ **Love your liver.** It helps metabolize fats and is a key organ for hormone regulation. A high-fat diet depletes liver function. A green tea combination, like Crystal Star's **GREEN TEA CLEANSER™**, (with green tea, gotu kola, fo-ti, and hawthorn) each morning can go a long way toward relieving liver congestion. Add **MILK THISTLE** extract if desired.

⇒ **Have a fresh salad every day.** Green leafy vegetables and whole grains are excellent sources of fiber, minerals and complex carbohydrates. They help stabilize blood sugar, reduce sugar craving, and are a good source of B vitamins.

⇒ **Vegetable protein is important because it stimulates the liver to clear estrogen metabolites**. It also seems to increase the length of time that progesterone stays in the body. Chinese studies show that soy-eating, vegetarian women eliminate more excess estrogen than meat eaters. Certain bacteria found in the colons of meat-eaters appear to actually synthesize estrogen, raising plasma estrogen levels.

⇒ **Essential fatty acids in your diet balance prostaglandins.**
Prostaglandins are vital, hormone-like compounds that act as transient hormones to regulate body functions almost like an electrical current. Foods like ocean fish, sea foods, olive, safflower, and sunflower oils, and herbs, such as evening primrose and flax oil, affect prostaglandin balance by supplementing and balancing the body's essential fatty acid supply. Too much saturated fat in the body, especially from meats and dairy products, inhibits both prostaglandin production and proper hormone flow. Arachidonic acid present in animal fats increases certain prostaglandins, which deplete progesterone levels and strain estrogen/progesterone ratios. Two to three 1000mg capsules of evening primrose oil daily, especially in conjunction with a broad spectrum herbal balancing compound, have shown excellent results for many women.

Does exercise help PMS? You bet it does! Regular exercise is a must for female balance. Aerobic, outdoor exercise is the best. We know it's hard to find time to add anything to your crowded day, but the benefits for controlling PMS are worth it. For PMS, exercise improves the way your body metabolizes hormones. It changes your food habits, and decreases craving for alcohol or tobacco. It makes you feel better by increasing levels of beta endorphins in the brain. It improves circulation to relieve congestion. It encourages regularity for rapid toxin elimination.

Relax more, too. Be sparing with your schedule during premenstrual days. Give yourself some slack, and take some time out to read, listen to music and relax. **Use stress reduction techniques.** Acupuncture and massage therapy are both effective as stress reduction techniques for PMS symptoms. Stretching/relaxation exercises such as yoga and tai chi help, too.

Daily self-massage of breasts and ovary areas relieves tension and relaxes reproductive organs. End your morning shower with a cool rinse to stimulate circulation and help relieve lymphatic congestion.

Note: Switch from tampons to pads if you are very congested.

Beyond diet and exercise, what are your best natural therapy choices for PMS? My first choices are balancing herbal compounds.

Phyto-hormone-rich herbal compounds to help balance estrogen levels. Phyto-estrogens are subtle and gentle, and remarkably similar to human hormones. They can help raise body estrogen levels when they are too low by stimulating the body's own hormone production.

Plant hormones can also help reduce excess body estrogen. At only $1/_{400th}$ to $1/_{50,000th}$ the strength of a woman's own circulating estrogens, phyto-estrogens are able to compete with human estrogens for receptor sites. When the weaker plant estrogens attach to the receptors, the net overall effect is a lowering of the body's estrogen levels, with obvious beneficial implications for excess-estrogen disease risks like breast and other hormone-driven cancers, and endometriosis.

Phytohormone-rich plants like soybeans and Mexican yams, and hormone-rich herbs like black cohosh, panax ginseng, licorice and dong quai, have a safety record of centuries. They offer a gentle, effective way to stimulate a woman's own body to produce amounts of estrogen and progesterone in the right proportion for her needs. In my experience, a combination of these herbs can be quite specific for PMS symptoms, especially when used in conjunction with **EVENING PRIMROSE OIL** over a two month menstrual cycle.

Broad-spectrum herbal combinations with these and other normalizing herbs, may be taken over a three to six month period as stabilizing resources for keeping the female system "very female."

A tea like **FEMALE HARMONY™** tea by Crystal Star with phyto-hormone-containing herbs, (*raspberry, licorice root, nettles, sarsaparilla, rose hips, spearmint and burdock*) may be used to relieve the physiological stress and emotional swings of PMS.

A phytohormone-rich formula like Crystal Star **FEMALE HARMONY™** capsules (with *dong quai, damiana, sarsaparilla and burdock roots, red raspberry, nettles, licorice root, dandelion* and more) may be used for PMS prevention over several months.

Note: Add two bayberry capsules if your flow is excessively heavy.

Many women's problems are thyroid involved. Iodine therapy from herbs and sea plants is a good place to look for PMS relief. Critical estrogen levels are controlled by thyroid hormones. Iodine is essential to thyroid gland health. If the thyroid does not receive enough iodine, insufficient thyroxine is produced and too much estrogen builds up. Balancing iodine for therapeutic results may be taken in from sea vegetables, at about 2 tablespoons daily in a soup or salad, or from iodine-containing herbs like those in **IODINE/POTASSIUM™** caps by Crystal Star, (with *kombu, kelp, dulse, spirulina, alfalfa, irish moss, watercress, borage and nettles*). Take with vitamin E for best absorption.

I also use SEA SEASONINGS by Maine Coast Sea Vegetables.

Adrenal insufficiency is common during PMS days, and it compounds the stress and fatigue experienced during this time. An herbal compound, like Crystal Star **ADR-ACTIVE™** (with *licorice root, sarsaparilla root, bladderwrack, uva ursi, rose hips, Irish moss, astragalus and ginger root*) can gently support adrenal function and raise energy without adding stimulants.

Bee products also provide adrenal support. I recommend Y.S. Farms ROYAL JELLY & GINSENG, and Beehive Botanicals FRESH POLLEN.

What about wild yam creams for PMS? They are in the news.... should they be a part of your PMS therapy program? Wild yam has a long herbal tradition as a balancer of women's estrogen and progesterone levels. Modern studies are conducting tests to see if wild yam can help alleviate PMS symptoms - especially in soothing nerves, lowering blood pressure and relieving cramping. Many women report that whole herb wild yam products exert a positive influence on PMS symptoms.

Some physicians today are prescribing *diosgenin,* a chemically modified phyto-sterol from wild yam under study. Diosgenin is being called "natural progesterone," because the molecular structure in the laboratory is the same as that made by the human body. There is controversy as to whether or not diosgenin converts into progesterone in the body.

In my experience, unprocessed **whole wild yam-based creams** show marked success for PMS symptoms. Acting transdermally as sources of plant progesterone, they offer many women estrogen/progesterone balance. The Crystal Star compound, **PRO-EST BALANCE™** gel. (with *wild yam, fresh American ginseng, licorice root, black cohosh, damiana and dong quai root among others, in a base of aloe vera, and grapeseed oil*) may be rolled on the abdomen area for relief.

Another specific herb, *Vitex,* *or* chaste tree berry, a 2000 year old herb, is widely used in Europe for women's menstrual disorders. Modern pharmacology tests show that vitex works through the pituitary gland, at a deep regulatory level, especially for PMS symptoms like depression, cramps, mood swings and menstrual water retention.

I have found, however, that *vitex works better when taken separately, as an adjunct* to herbal compounds like **PRO-EST BALANCE™**, or **FEMALE HARMONY™**. The 1-2% of cases reporting side effects, reported them when *vitex was included within the herbal combination instead of taken separately.* Vitex is a nourishing herb that slowly, gently creates a fundamental change in the cyclic hormonal balance. Vitex should be taken long-term for optimum effects. It may take ten days for noticeable results; optimum benefits may take up to six months or longer.

Which products should you buy? In addition to the Crystal Star Herbal Nutrition formulas listed earlier, there are many fine hormone balancing compounds for women in health food stores today. Here are some we have tested and found effective.

- REJUVENATE FOR WOMEN by Golden Pride
- Biochem Formula PRE-MENSES P.M.S. by Country Life.
- PMS FORTE and HERBAL HARMONY by Futurebiotics
- WOMEN'S PHASE 1 by Transitions For Health
- FEM-CARE™ by Enzymatic Therapy
- PRO-GEST BODY CREAM by Transitions
- WILD YAM MOISTURIZING CREME by Premier
- PHYTO-SPROUT PLUS - a soy complex by Healthy Tek
- FEMALE FORMULA, a nourishing tonic used in rotation with PMS HERBAL by Zand Herbal Formulas.

Can you address specific PMS problems with natural therapy?
We've talked about diet and hormone balance as foundation therapy for PMS, but beyond this overall, holistic help, women can also use very directed programs for their individual problems. Herbs in particular, can be highly specific to pinpoint particular body needs.

We'll consider some of the most commonly experienced problems.

❧**Abdominal Pain and Cramping** involves several common conditions, the most usual being pelvic congestion and/or inflammation, spasmodic pain caused by uterine contractions, and pre-menstrual muscle contractions expressed in shooting pains that radiate from the lower abdomen to the back and thighs.

About ten days before menstruation begins, the level of calcium in the blood begins to drop and continues to drop until about three days into the cycle. Blood calcium deficiency can cause muscle cramping, headaches, water retention, achiness, depression and insomnia.

❧ Effective herbal therapies:
Herbs offer relief from menstrual cramping, by relaxing muscles and easing uterine contractions.

1) Crystal Star has an effective, anti-spasmodic combination - **ANTI-SPZ™** (with cramp bark, black haw, rosemary, kava kava, passionflower, wild yam, St. John's wort and raspberry.

2) A strong muscle relaxing herbal combination for cramps might look the **CRAMP BARK COMBO™** by Crystal Star, (with cramp bark, rosemary, black haw, kava kava and lobelia)

3) Cramping may also be swiftly alleviated with a topical, plant-derived progesterone cream, applied several times daily. (See Crystal Star **PRO-EST BALANCE™** on page 12 for formula.)

Increase calcium intake about ten days prior to the period to insure an adequate supply of blood calcium. Focus on foods like sesame seeds, yogurt, sea vegetables, sprouts, dark green leafy vegetables, and herbs such as comfrey, raspberry and nettles.

• Take an herbal calcium supplement like Crystal Star **CALCIUM SOURCE™** or FLORADIX CALCIUM by Flora, Inc.

• Chamomile tea may be used for mild cramping. For more severe cramps, use white willow extract or Crystal Star ANTI-FLAM™.

• Take **EVENING PRIMROSE oil** for several months to balance prostaglandins, which are often responsible for uterine cramping.

⅊Headaches, Depression and Mood Swings go hand in hand for many women during menstruation.

St. John's Wort is receiving a great deal of publicity today as an effective **herbal anti-depressant.** Many naturopaths also recommend it for PMS-related mood swings. Components in St. John's Wort alter brain chemistry in a way which improves mood. A recent clinical study on women with PMS-involved depression showed that St. John's Wort improved symptoms of anxiety, depression, and low confidence, and greatly improved sleep quality. I find that St. John's Wort works far better in combination with other synergistic herbs than alone.

⅊ Effective herbal therapies:

A fast-acting combination, **DEPRESSEX™** (with St. John's wort, kava kava,, Am. ginseng, Ayurvedic ashwagandha, gotu kola, rosemary, Siberian ginseng, fo-ti and wood betony) has been notably successful at easing stress, tension, mood swings and anxiety.

• HARMONY by Transitions is an effective formula for depression and mood swings. It calms nerves and levels emotions.

• A simple herbal tea, **FLOW EASE™** by Crystal Star, (with cramp bark, angelica, squaw vine, chamomile, sarsaparilla and ginger,) can do much to relax stress and ease muscle tension.

• A soothing combination for PMS headaches is Crystal Star **ANTI-FLAM™**, (with white willow, St. John's wort, echinacea root, white pine bark, gotu kola, chamomile, alfalfa and red clover blsm., among others). It helps reduce swelling and inflammation and may be used much as aspirin is used without the irritation.

I also recommend boosting your body's B-vitamins with a Vitamin B complex (50 mg, three times a day); and adding a calcium/magnesium supplement, in equal proportions (500mg, four times daily) to alleviate muscle tension.

⅊Unusual Fatigue and Lack of Energy as symptoms of PMS are often the result of exhausted adrenal glands. Herbal combinations can provide adrenal support without adding stimulants or raw animal glandular tissue. A simple combination like **ADR-ACTIVE™** from Crystal Star, (with *licorice root, bladderwrack, sarsaparilla - a specific for adrenal fatigue - and Irish moss), also* encourages adrenal cortex production, improving other PMS conditions, such as skin problems at the same time.

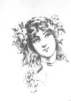

❧ Effective adrenal gland herbal therapies:

• Take Crystal Star **ADR-ACTIVE™** formula (previous page) with **BODY REBUILDER™** caps (with *spirulina, bee pollen, alfalfa, rosehips vitamin C, hawthorn, barley grass, Siberian ginseng* and *sarsaparilla*).

• **Add a green superfood supplement, such as Crystal Star SYSTEMS STRENGTH™,** a potent vegetarian blend of superfoods like *soy protein, miso, cranberry juice* and *acidolphilus,* sea vegetables like *spirulina, dulse, wakame, kombu* and *chlorella,* and herbal heavyweights like *barley grass, Siberian ginseng, licorice rt., pau d'arco, schizandra* and *alfalfa* to strengthen the body's systems.

or a superfood like Wakunaga KYO-GREEN drink.

• **Ginseng is an adrenal specific.** Consider **GINSENG SIX™ Super Energy Caps** by Crystal Star, a blend of six of the world's most potent ginsengs, (like *panax, Siberian, Chinese kirin, suma* and *tienchi*); or • WILD AMERICAN GINSENG by HSU's Ginseng Ent., or • ginseng with high potency royal jelly, or • SIBERIAN GINSENG extract under the tongue twice daily.

• Adrenal balancing teas include licorice root ginseng/licorice root, gotu kola, hawthorn leaf, berry and flower tea.

❧ **Pre-Period Edema, Water Retention and Body Heaviness** are the result of metabolism as well as hormonal changes. The body slightly alters the way it processes salts and carbohydrates during pre-menstrual days, leaving women feeling bloated and heavy. A low progesterone-to-estrogen ratio can cause the PMS symptoms of bloating, irritability and depression. Excessive fluid retention is a main cause of the congestive symptoms seen with cramps that are characterized by dull, aching pain.

We know that constant use of chemical diuretics leaches potassium through the urine, and leads to other body imbalances. **Do diuretic herbs do the same thing?** Even though any herbal formula may be taken to excess, diuretic herbs or a gentle diuretic tea like Crystal Star **TINKLE TEA™** (with herbs like *uva ursi, senna leaf, fennel seed, dandelion* and *parsley,* among others) are in the main, body balancers, helping the body to flush out **excess fluid,** rather than too much fluid. I recommend eating foods that are high in potassium such as bananas, oranges, broccoli, nuts and seeds, and most fruits. Potassium has a diuretic effect on the body tissues and helps reduce bloating.

Green tea each morning during your pre-period also cleanses excess fluid and provides a quick, easy mini-detox.

⅋Breast Swelling and Soreness are signs of body congestion. Relieving breast tenderness may be accomplished by daily diet techniques.

> ### ⅋ Effective: natural therapies:
> A daily six capsule regimen for breast soreness symptoms: 1 B Complex 100mg, 1 vitamin C with bioflavonoids 1000mg, 1 brome-lain 500mg. 2x daily, and 2 **EVENING PRIMROSE oil** 500mg.
> • For prevention therapy, use DANDELION EXTRACT or TEA.
> • Vitamin E also relieves breast swelling and soreness. In one study, 400IU daily were given for 3 months to women with breast tenderness. Most had moderate to complete relief of discomfort. The women with breast cysts noted reduction in the size of the cysts.

⅋Delayed or Suppressed Menstruation when you are not pregnant is another sign of body congestion, and probably adrenal gland imbalance as well. In young girls, menses may be delayed because of low estrogen secretion due to low blood calcium levels. A menstrual cycle may be delayed or stop altogether due to a lack of protein in the diet. (If you are an athlete, be especially certain that there is an adequate supply of good-quality protein in your diet.)

> ### ⅋ Effective: natural therapies:
> A Crystal Star phyto-estrogen **FEM-SUPPORT™** blend (*dong quai, damiana* and *ashwagandha*), especially when taken with a cup of *burdock tea*, is effective in stimulating the estrogen cycle.
> • In addition, 4 to 6 **EVENING PRIMROSE oil** capsules daily, along with **VITEX** extract, and a regular calcium, magnesium and zinc supplement, can help balance prostaglandin formation.
>
> • If you have "marathoners syndrome," intensive body building and sports training that suppresses menses, because body fat, and therefore estrogen levels, become extremely reduced. The body does not slough off endometrial tissue when it feels at risk in being able to form more. Women who train for competition sometimes experience total cessation of menses.
> • Eat plenty of iron and calcium rich foods. Increase Omega-3 fatty acids like flax oil; and take an herbal hormone balancing formula like Crystal Star **FEMALE HARMONY™** for 3 to 6 months.

👑**Mouth Sores and Facial Blemishes** are signs of temporary hormone imbalance.

✵ Effective: natural therapies:

Topical skin healing herbs are effective for trouble spots - like Crystal Star's **BEAUTIFUL SKIN™ Gel,** (with extracts of *licorice root, burdock root, rosemary, rose hips, sarsaparilla, sage, chamomile, thyme, dandelion, royal jelly, ginseng and aloe vera.*

• Crystal Star's **BEAUTIFUL SKIN™ Tea** with many of the same herbs, may be used both topically and internally for outstanding results in skin therapy.

• A simple herbal preventive for herpes-type mouth sores is Crystal Star **LYSINE-LICORICE HEALING™ Gel**, (with extra extracts of *myrrh, grapefruit seed and aloe vera*).

Also consider:
• HERPANACINE by Dr. Wayne Diamond - an extremely effective skin healer that often works when nothing else is effective.
• HERPILYN by Enzymatic Therapy - a medicated cream for cold sores and fever blisters.

👑**Excessive Menstrual Flow and Spotting** usually occurs because low levels of progesterone result in tissue build up. Progesterone is the hormone factor that controls uniform shedding of the uterine lining during menstruation. If at the same time, a woman has relatively high levels of estrogen that stimulate the uterine lining, a great deal of endometrial tissue is formed. The combination of the two factors leads to abnormally heavy flow during menstruation, and/or spotting between periods as excess tissue is shed.

A good diet is important to normalize flow. Women who eat a nutrient-poor diet are also at high risk of heavy menstrual bleeding because they lack the nutrients to regulate normal blood flow. Studies show that deficiencies of vitamin A, vitamin C, iron, and bioflavonoids worsen or even cause heavy menstrual bleeding. Include plenty of vegetables, fruits and high-quality vegetable protein in your diet. Iodine is significant. Include sea vegetables in the diet for high-quality trace minerals. Avoid problem foods like white sugar, salty snacks, fried foods, and caffeine.

A high fat diet also encourages excess estrogen. Too much fat, especially from dairy foods, may cause the uterine lining to thicken releasing heavy, painful menstrual flow.

❧ Effective: natural therapies:

Look for formulas with two herbs traditionally used to stop excessive menstrual flow and postparum hemorrhaging - goldenseal and shepherd's purse. Goldenseal contains berberine that calms uterine muscular tension. Shepherd's purse helps promote blood clotting and is used to help stop menstrual bleeding

• A hemostatic combination that aids fat metabolism by the liver, has citrus bioflavs to strengthen tissue and reduce capillary fragility, and encourages prostaglandin balance would include *shepherd's purse, white oak, oatstraw, bayberry, burdock, borage seed, dulse, goldenseal, nettles, lemon and milk thistle seed.*

• Add 2 *bayberry* caps and Futurebiotics PHYTO-FLAVONOIDS - a concentrated flavonoid fromula with grape extract, or WOMEN'S SELECT by Matrix Health if menstruation is extremely heavy.

• Once flow has lessened, take a broad-based female harmonizing formula like Crystal Star **FEMALE HARMONY™** (with *dong quai, damiana, sarsaparilla, burdock, raspberry, rosemary, nettles, dandelion and licorice root* among others),for the next 2 to 3 months to normalize hormone production.

Excessive menstrual flow means iron deficiency for many women. Women with this condition have a great deal of fatigue from heavy blood loss during menstruation. An iron-rich herbal combination, like Crystal Star's **IRON SOURCE™** (with herbs like *alfalfa, beet root, dandelion, yellow dock, parsley and Siberian ginseng*) can work as a hemoglobin builder for better absorption of iron and minerals. It also encourages increased spleen and liver activity for better red blood cell production and tissue oxygen.

• A similar formula by *RASPBERRY/NETTLES by* master herbalist Rosemary Gladstar has measureable amounts of naturally occurring calcium and iron.

Menstruation is a natural part of a woman's life. PMS is not. Women can take control of PMS naturally and effectively.

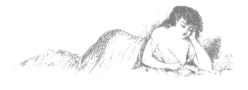

Endometriosis Responds To Natural Therapies

Endometriosis is a complex problem. Eight to ten million American women between the ages of 25 and 40 experience this extremely painful, inflamed gynecological condition. It is caused by mislocation and overgrowth of uterine endometrial tissue, and attachment of this tissue to other organs. It is normal tissue growing in abnormal places, sometimes spreading as far as the lungs. The endometrial fragments are functioning tissue and therefore bleed every month just as if they were still in the uterus and part of the normal menstrual cycle. Much of the waste blood flows back through the fallopian tubes or the rectum instead of normally through the vagina. Endometriosis is not life-threatening, but it significantly increases risk for uterine and breast fibroids.

Why is it so hard to diagnose? Endometriosis is difficult to diagnose because there are no external symptoms. It is mysterious because, even though migratory endometrial cells frequently appear outside the uterus during menstruation, they only develop into endometriosis in some women. Indicators for women who develop endometriosis are high levels of estrogen, deficient progesterone, overall hormone imbalance, the presence of sexually transmitted viruses (such as chlamydia and condyloma acuminata) prostaglandin imbalance from magnesium and essential fatty acid deficiency, and hypoglycemia.

New theories blame endometriosis on a glitch in the immune system. Naturopaths see good results when they treat endometriosis as an immune deficient disease.

What are the symptoms? How do you know if you have it?
The typical profile for endometriosis is recurring, severe cramping with extreme abdominal and rectal pain during menses and ovulation, and unusually heavy vaginal and rectal bleeding during menstruation. Women with endometriosis have painful, prolonged periods. There is also pelvic pain during intercourse, fluid retention, swelling of the abdomen and abdominal bleeding, irritable bowel syndrome and gas, nerve pain, and insomnia. Endometriosis often results in infertility.

Traditional medical approach relies on hormone-suppressing drugs and surgery. Because of the hormone connection, and since at very low estrogen levels (which preclude a woman from having a menstrual cycle), the endometrial tissue doesn't grow or bleed, medical therapy for endometriosis concentrates on altering a woman's hormone level with estrogen, or birth control pills, and suppressing menstruation with drugs.

While some of the drugs have been successful in relieving the symptoms of endometriosis, each one has notable, unpleasant side effects, including acne, bloating, and male characteristics like decreased breast size and facial hair growth. Before you jump into surgery or any drastic treatment decision, endometrial fibroids often go away when glands and hormones rebalance, such as after pregnancy and childbirth, or after menopause when estrogen levels drop. Avoid low dose birth control pills for endometriosis. Call 1-800-992-ENDO for up-to-date support.

Diet improvement helps control symptoms. Studies show, and I personally know women with endometriosis who report a noticeable decrease in heavy bleeding and pain levels within one or two menstrual cycles after starting an optimum diet program. In fact, no therapy can be fully effective without diet improvement as part of the treatment plan.

1. Lower your fat intake to reduce body fat and excess circulating estrogen. It's the single most effective change you can make in your diet to prevent endometriosis. Endometriosis symptoms are aggravated too much dietary fat, and its a clear cause of over production of estrogen. Especially avoid *saturated* fat from red meats, (which may also have injected hormones). Excessive saturated fat stresses your liver, too, making it less able to break down estrogen efficiently, leading to excess estrogen levels. Avoid hard-to-digest hydrogenated oils. Use flax oil instead of butter, and small amounts of oils like olive oil or canola oil for cooking or stir-frying. Low fat poultry meat is ok, (but may also be injected with hormones). Look for "yard-raised" or "free-range" poultry. Avoid full fat dairy foods, and high fat nuts and seeds to reduce your fat.

2. Reduce sugary foods of all kinds, (including sugary alcoholic drinks), because they affect the way your body processes fats. Sugar, like alcohol depletes the body's B vitamins and minerals, which can worsen both muscle and nerve tension, irritability and anxiety.

However, sufficient *essential fatty acids* are extremely important for a woman's body, especially if she has menstrual cramping caused by endometriosis or fibroid tumors. Fatty acids are the raw materials from which the important hormone-like chemicals called prostaglandins are made. Prostaglandins have muscle and blood-vessel-relaxant properties that can significantly reduce muscle cramps, tension and painful pelvic symptoms. Dietary essential fatty acids (Omega-6 and Omega-3 families) are found primarily in seeds, like flax and sesame, nuts like almonds, and fish like salmon, mackerel and trout.

3. Eliminate caffeine in all forms (especially coffee and chocolate) from your diet. Caffeine increases anxiety, irritability and mood swings. It also depletes body stores of B-complex vitamins and essential minerals. Studies show long term use of caffeine can increase endometriosis-related pain, cramps, and bleeding by disrupting both carbohydrate metabolism and healthy liver function.

4. Eliminate or reduce dairy products in your diet. Dairy products are the main dietary source of arachidonic acid, the fat used by your body to produce muscle-contracting F_2 Alpha prostaglandins. These prostaglandins can increase pelvic pain, cramps, and inflammation. The high saturated fat content of dairy products is a risk factor for excess estrogen levels in the body.

5. Eat vegetables to control endometriosis - especially a large green salad every day. Studies show that vegetarian women eating a low fat, high fiber diet release two to three times more estrogen in their bowel movements and have 50 percent lower blood levels of estrogen than women eating a diet high in dairy and animal fats. Vegetables high in calcium, magnesium and potassium help relieve and prevent cramps, calming emotions as well as muscles. Vitamin C in vegetables and fruits also helps reduce heavy menstrual flow, prevents capillary fragility and promotes good circulation to tense pelvic muscles.

6. Soy foods can be a "best bet" for endometriosis. Soy foods like tofu, tempeh and miso help regulate body estrogen levels because soy is a rich source of plant estrogens and flavonoids that have a chemical structure similar to human estrogen, but much weaker in potency. Soy estrogens help lower human estrogen levels by interfering with excess estrogen production and reducing bleeding problems.

➤ **The goal is to keep your body chemistry alkaline.**
- **Alkalizing foods to eat** during healing include all vegetables and sea vegetables, most fruits, and soy foods like tofu and miso.
- **Acid forming foods to restrict** during healing include red meats, eggs, cheese, sugar, and all saturated fats, because they produce F_2 Alpha prostaglandins that trigger muscle contraction, inflammation and constriction in blood vessels, worsening endometriosis-related cramps and the spread of endometrial implants. Note: Too much salt has the same effects, and contributes to bloating. Use seasonings like garlic, herbs, spices and lemon juice instead.

A diet that boosts the immune system is critical. Take a "green drink" from dark green leafy vegetables, sea vegetables and blue/green algae at least twice a week during healing. You can make a fresh one from scratch, using a recipe from my book **COOKING FOR HEALTHY HEALING** Or use Crystal Star's **ENERGY GREEN™** Drink (with superfoods like *barley grass, alfalfa, Siberian ginseng, chlorella, dulse, oats and spirulina*). Other good green superfoods include Nutricology PRO-GREENS, Green Foods GREEN MAGMA, KYO-GREEN by Wakunaga, EASY GREENS by Transitions, and BEST OF GREENS or GREEN KAMUT by Green Kamut.

Herbal medicines are a key part of natural therapy for endometriosis because they can help reduce inflammation, balance estrogen/progesterone ratios, and boost immune strength. Herbal therapy programs also address liver performance, improve emotional stress and relieve pain. Herbs are gentle, effective remedies with hormone-balancing effects that help lower excessive estrogen levels and control heavy bleeding.

Some herbs provide additional sources of essential nutrients, like calcium, magnesium and potassium that help relieve painful symptoms.

Herbal bioflavonoids help control endometriosis and fibroids. Bioflavonoids are both estrogenic and anti-estrogenic, important properties for control of endometriosis and fibroid symptoms. Good sources of bioflavonoids include hawthorn berries, citrus fruits, bilberries, grape skins, cherries and red clover.

Here is a three month herbal program to reduce inflammation, increase progesterone levels, and balance prostaglandins:

For the first month:
• Take eight 500mg **EVENING PRIMROSE OIL** capsules daily.
• Drink two cups of BURDOCK TEA daily.
• Take up to 10,000mg. ascorbate vitamin C daily. Decrease dosage when the stool turns soupy.
* Take six capsules daily of **WOMEN'S BEST FRIEND™** Caps by Crystal Star. It contains herbs like *goldenseal root, cramp bark, squaw vine, red raspberry, dong quai, sarsaparilla, false unicorn, peony and rose hips* with anti-biotic, anti-inflammatory properties.

Follow with a tissue healing program the next month:
• Take two cups daily of **WOMAN'S STRENGTH ENDO™** Tea by Crystal Star (with *dandelion root, wild yam, sarsaparilla, burdock root, pau d'arco bark, chaste tree berry and milk thistle seed*)
* BLACK COHOSH EXTRACT to dissolve abnormally placed tissue.
* DANDELION ROOT extract to help metabolize excess estrogen.

• **SHARK LIVER OIL** capsules as an anti-infective.
• Gently detoxify and stimulate the liver to metabolize estrogen with **BITTERS & LEMON**™ by Crystal Star (with *Oregon grape root, cardamom seed, gentian root, senna, dandelion and peppermint*) Don't take during painful flare-up
• Extra **VITEX EXTRACT** 2x daily.
• **GRAPE SEED EXTRACT** by NutriCology to prevent release and synthesis of compounds that promote inflammation.

Follow with a rebuilding, healing program to reduce excess estrogen levels and regulate hormone production:
• Take two cups daily of the following tea: **WOMAN'S STRENGTH ENDO**™ Tea by Crystal Star. (see previous month's program) or Solgar **ISO SOY** (*soy protein / isoflavone concentrated phyto-hormone-rich powder*)
• **BLACK COHOSH EXTRACT** to dissolve abnormally placed tissue.
• **DANDELION ROOT** extract to help metabolize excess estrogen.
• Rebuild liver tissue with **MILK THISTLE SEED EXTRACT**, or **DANDELION/ BURDOCK FORMULA** - a Rosemary Gladstar formula of digestive bitters to support normal liver function.

Is there anything natural I can do for the pain?
Herbs can help reduce pain and inflammation. Strong herbal analgesics relax pelvic muscles and relieve contractions. Crystal Star **CRAMP BARK COMBO**™ extract (with *cramp bark, black cohosh, valerian, wild yam, white willow and licorice*) may generally be used as needed.

• I also recommend an accompanying adrenal gland support formula, like Crystal Star **ADR-ACTIVE**™ (with herbs like *licorice root, sarsaparilla root, bladderwrack and Irish moss*) along with **EVENING PRIMROSE OIL** twice a day for best results:

Once again, as in all natural healing programs, immune enhancement is the key to permanent results.
• Add a sea plant source of beta carotene like Solgar's OCEAN CAROTENE caps, CoQ_{10}, 60mg 3 times daily, Ester C with bioflavonoids, 3000mg daily, and vitamin E 800IU daily to boost immunity.
• **Add a non-constipating, easy to take herbal iron, like** Crystal Star IRON SOURCE™ (with herbs like *beet root, yellow dock, dulse, dandelion, parsley, borage and alfalfa*) if bleeding has been very heavy.

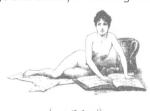

Plant-derived wild yam creams are big news today. Are they a source of progesterone? Should you add them to your program for endometriosis?

First, let's unravel some of the mystery about progesterone.

Progesterone, along with estrogen, is one of two main hormones made by a woman's ovaries. It is also made in smaller amounts by the adrenal glands. Progesterone participates in almost every physiological process, and is a precursor of other steroid hormones made by the body.

As far back as in the 1950's, active estrogen and progesterone-like substances were identified in many plants, especially the wild yam. Called phyto-estrogens and phyto-progesterones, it was discovered that these natural substances could be used inexpensively to create synthetic, patentable variations of progesterone (progestins). However, the altered structure of the synthetic varieties, meant that they worked outside the body's normal hormone and enzyme pathways. Side effects quickly appeared, from headaches to bloating, weight gain, *and* an increased risk of breast and uterine tumors. Most physicians were not educated about the difference between natural progesterone and synthetic progestins.

Today, there are three categories of progesterone:

1) Synthetic progesterone - man-made hormones that are patentable progesterone analogs made from yam-derived natural progesterone. These progestational agents are referred to as progestins, progestogens and gestagens, all meaning "a synthetically derived compound with the ability to sustain the human secretory endometrium."

2) Synthesized progesterone from plant saponins - converted under hydrolyzation to sapogenins, of which two (sarsasapogenin, from sarsaparilla, and diosgenin, from wild yam) are the main sterol sources for the so-called natural progesterone in medical use. Controversy about wild yam's effectiveness stems from whether diosgenin, the substance derived from wild yam, converts into progesterone in a woman's body. While there has been no modern, double-blind accredited study that currently exists proving or disproves progesterone action, wild yam products clearly appear to exert progesterone-like effects in normalizing a woman's hormone balance. **This is the type of progesterone found in many progesterone creams on the market.**

3) **Whole plant** wild yam herbal formulas - which contain phyto-progesterones and the full spectrum of complementary, protective plant constituents naturally inherent in the plant. Whole plant wild yam is body balancing with restorative effects for both woman and men.

A study of the Trobriand islanders near New Guinea, showed that they have a diet dedicated to yams with the sterol diosgenin, (and its progesterone-like effects). While they eat other vegetables, fruit and fish. the wild yam is their cultural symbol of life and good health for the islanders, who believe that people who eat plenty of yams are generally slim, happy, enjoy excellent health and have a vigorous sex life.

So, although wild yam testing is more recent for endometriosis than for PMS or osteoporosis, many naturopaths are concluding that whole wild yam creams do play a role in balancing estrogen/progesterone levels and in reducing abnormal cell growth. Crystal Star has a roll-on formula called **PRO-EST BALANCE™**, (with *aloe vera, grapeseed oil, extracts of wild yam, fresh American ginseng, dong quai, licorice root, black cohosh, burdock and sarsaparilla root*), that has shown good empirical observation results.

NOTE: Check out the next section on Breast and Uterine Fibroids, too. It includes suggestions for fibroids that also apply for endometriosis.

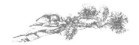

Natural Therapies Help Reduce Breast and Uterine Fibroids

Disheartening new statistics show that 1 of every 1500 women in America between the ages of 35 and 49 are struggling with fibroid breast growths. One of every five women over the age of thirty has a uterine fibroid tumor or myomata. Already the most common type of tumor occurring in the body, the risk of fibroids increases dramatically with age. By age 75, about 1 of every 230 women has fibroids.

What are fibroids? How do you know if you have them?

Breast fibroids are moveable, benign nodules or cysts near the surface of the breasts. We know that an estrogen imbalance is involved, because they usually go away when menopause begins and the body's estrogen secretions naturally reduce.

The breast lumps fluctuate in extent, from barely detectable to the size of a golf ball sometimes becoming painfully inflamed. They are normally in phase with the menstrual cycle.

During each menstrual cycle, there is stimulation of the breast hormones. Breast fibroids apparently develop due to an imbalanced estrogen-to-progesterone ratio. As hormone levels fall after menses, the breasts return to their prestimulation size and function. In many women these changes are so slight that symptoms do not appear, but for others, significant inflammation occurs.

Breast fibroids are not cancer, and have little chance of becoming cancerous. However, because of their body chemistry characteristics, breast cancer does occur more frequently in women with fibroids.

New fibroid growths that occur after menopause, may be a sign of breast cancer, and should be attended to immediately.

Remember, though, that **fibroid lumps are not fixed, like *breast cancer* lumps,** but can be moved around freely.

Uterine Fibroids:

Less than one-half of one percent of all fibroid tumors become cancerous. But they still cause a wide range of other problems, especially pressure and pain on nearby organs. One-third of all hysterectomies are performed on women suffering pain, excessive bleeding or other complications due to fibroids. Almost 50 percent of women with fibroids develop severe symptoms that benefit from medical intervention. Surgery is not the only solution, although it may be necessary for women with very large and painful fibroids. Alternative therapies work best at reducing painful symptoms and may be used as preventive measures.

Uterine fibroids, unlike cancer, do not spread, remaining within the confines of the uterus, but they can develop in different areas of the uterus - extending into the uterine cavity from the endometrium, within the uterine walls, or on the outside of the uterus in the lining between the uterus and the pelvic cavity. They may grow within the uterine muscle or may protrude into the uterine cavity and remain attached to the wall. Significant growth of fibroids can cause the entire uterus, and therefore the abdomen, to enlarge as if a woman were pregnant.

What causes fibroids? Why are they becoming so prevalent?

The medical community sees fibroids as another case where early detection is the answer. The usual scenario is:

1) early detection through mammograms
2) followed by a surgical biopsy
3) followed by surgery to remove the fibroid.

The natural healing world sees fibroids as a result of body chemistry imbalances...sometimes brought on by the very mammograms used to detect them!

There is a very real risk in receiving regular doses of radiation through mammograms, even though the dosage is less than that received in the 1970's and 80's. Breast tissue is so sensitive and delicate that the time between a mammogram and fibroid growth is sometimes as little as three months. I feel that unless a person is at high risk for breast cancer, discovery methods should center on breast self-exams, with mammograms reserved for confirming a doctor's diagnosis.

Besides the harm X-rays can do, the tests themselves are often inaccurate, with **15% false negatives and 30% false positives**. The attendant invasive medical procedures are painful. Many women are turning to alternative methods to reduce breast fibroids. Natural therapies have been consistently successful in helping a woman avoid surgery and return her body to natural balance. Thyroid imbalance, primarily an underactive thyroid, is also involved, (a problem for many people born after WW II), as well as too much dietary fat, which stores excess hormones.

If you are taking estrogen replacement therapy, ask your doctor about studies indicating that ERT keeps fibroids growing even after menopause.

Breast fibroids are much more sensitive to estrogen stimulation than normal tissue. Women approaching menopause, and those with high estrogen levels due to pregnancy or certain birth control pills are more susceptible to them. Women who have a family history of fibroids and who eat a high-fat diet are also at risk. A diet high in fat and low in fiber prevents the liver from breaking down estrogen into less potent chemical forms; it also slows down normal estrogen release so that it tends to reabsorb back into the bloodstream.

Uterine fibroids generally shrink when estrogen influence is low, such as the post-partum period and after a menstrual period, but they resume growth when estrogen levels rise again. They often stop growing, and even shrink, after menopause. Unfortunately, for some post-menopausal women, the use of estrogen replacement therapy may reactivate and stimulate the fibroid growth, one of the worst side effects of synthetic hormones. A low fat diet and herbal supplement plan that manages estrogen levels, as well as alternative options to estrogen replacement therapy can help keep fibroids under control.

What symptoms should alert you to the presence of fibroids?

Symptoms are not always be apparent; many women have fibroids for years and don't feel any discomfort. About 50% experience severe symptoms. The most common problems are heavy menstrual bleeding and inter-period spotting, pelvic pressure and pain, unusual urinary frequency, chronic constipation, hemorrhoids, infertility and a high risk of miscarriage. Many symptoms can be managed through diet and lifestyle improvement.

About one-third of women with fibroids suffer from abnormal uterine bleeding. Many also develop a heavier menstrual flow that often lasts longer than normal. Most experience bleeding between periods. This type of abnormal bleeding occurs when the fibroids grow into the uterine cavity, expanding the cavity area by 10 to 15 times - and providing a greater surface area on which to bleed each month. Fibroids also press against uterine blood vessels disrupting normal blood flow. If the fibroids grow in the wall of the uterus, they restrict uterine contractions and interfere with the elasticity of the endometrial blood vessels, resulting in excessive menstrual bleeding.

The high estrogen levels often present in women with fibroids can disrupt normal functioning of the uterine lining. The balance between estrogen and progesterone normally regulates the amount of blood loss, but when estrogen levels are elevated, blood loss from the endometrium increases and adds to the excessive flow already caused by the fibroids.

Many women with fibroids experience pelvic pressure and pain, largely due to the growing fibroids. A fibroid pressing against the bladder can cause a reduction in bladder capacity, resulting in frequent urination and urgency. Occasionally, this pressure may even lead to kidney damage. Fibroids that press on the bowels may cause constipation or hemorrhoids.

Fibroids may be the cause of as much as 10% of infertility cases. They can inhibit implantation of the fertilized egg in the uterine lining, or compress the fallopian tube or disrupt the lining of the uterus. Fibroids may cause miscarriage, especially during the first trimester of pregnancy, by pressing upon the uterine cavity, or by altering the blood flow that would normally nourish the growing fetus.

New studies show that **stress may play an underlying role in the formation of fibroids.** Here's why.

Women today contend with many emotional and social changes: career choices, marital issues, and feelings of having lost their youth. Stresses like these may suppress ovulation, thus raising estrogen levels and encouraging a favorable climate for fibroids. Under severe stress, a woman may produce only estrogen during the menstrual cycle, instead of the normal combination of estrogen and progesterone. Relaxation techniques like deep breathing, yoga stretches, a daily walk, and positive visualization help alleviate anxiety, and also help stabilize estrogen levels.

What lifestyle steps can you take to prevent fibroids?
Most experts agree that fibroids are not inherited, but seem to be dependent on lifestyle and environment. I believe that prevention is largely a matter of lifestyle decisions.

Here is a THREE-POINT PREVENTION PROGRAM that has been used effectively by thousands of women.
A) Make diet changes to guard against fibroid formation:
• Lower the fat in your diet to 20% or less of your calorie intake. Fats stimulate estrogen uptake, excess estrogen retention and salt retention.

• Eliminate fried foods, especially during your menstrual cycle.

• Minimize intake of caffeine. There is a definite correlation.

• Follow a largely vegetarian diet to help keep estrogen levels in line. Minimize or avoid meat and dairy products that regularly contain hormones, like red meats, fatty dairy foods and commercial poultry. (*Note: Foster Farms poultry and Diestal Turkeys Farms say they do not use hormones on their birds.*)

• Reduce high-stress foods like animal products, alcohol and sugar that overwork the liver, leaving it unable to break down estrogen efficiently. (Note: although most whole grain foods are beneficial, women with severe fibroid symptoms may need to avoid whole wheat. Wheat contains gluten protein which is difficult to digest and can be allergenic. If you have a gluten intolerance, it may worsen fatigue, depression, bloating, constipation, diarrhea and intestinal cramps.

B) Take phyto-hormone-rich herbal combinations to lower the amount of circulating estrogen in the body and reduce inflammation.
• Take an herbal formula to prevent or retard fibroid growth, like Crystal Star's WOMAN'S BALANCE FIBRO™ caps, (with *pau d' arco, burdock, goldenseal, black cohosh, dandelion, dong quai, licorice root and ashwagandha*).

• Add EVENING PRIMROSE oil daily to reduce inflammation.

C) Keep your liver and thyroid gland strong.
• The body gets rid of excess estrogen in the liver. If the liver is weak, estrogen accumulates allowing problems like fibroids and endometriosis. Today's assault of environmental, pseudo and synthetic estrogens greatly taxes the liver.

• Add a B complex supplement and sea vegetables to your daily program.

Can you reduce or eliminate fibroids?

Here is the FOUR POINT PROGRAM I use:

A) Make important diet improvements:

• **Avoid caffeine-containing foods**, and foods that leach magnesium, like carbonated drinks.

• **Add iodine and potassium-rich foods**, like miso, and sea vegetables to balance your thyroid activity.

• **Add soy foods to your diet**. They help regulate and lower estrogen levels in the body. Soy plant estrogens are remarkably similar to human circulating estrogens - so much so that they can compete with the body's estrogen in binding to human estrogen receptors. Yet, since plant estrogens are extremely subtle, (only $1/_{50,000}$ the potency of synthetic estrogen), our receptor cell uptake of these instead of other estrogens helps block too much estrogen production, a clear factor in fibroids and breast tumors. Soy foods have also been found to help reduce bleeding problems in premenopausal women with fibroid tumors.

• **Add mineral-rich legumes** like beans, peas, black beans, chickpeas, lentils, pinto and lima beans. Legumes contain highly absorbable calcium, magnesium, potassium, iron, copper and zinc. Women with fibroids and endometriosis who suffer from heavy bleeding are often deficient in these minerals. Calcium and magnesium help decrease menstrual pain, discomfort and irritability. Potassium helps relieve the symptoms of menstrual congestion by reducing fluid retention and bloating. Non-constipating, vegetable iron helps reduce bleeding and cramps. Legumes are also high in vitamin B complex nutrients for healthy liver function, (which helps reduce excess estrogen levels) and helps prevent menstrual cramps.

• **Eat more vegetables for fiber.** Vegetable fiber foods bind to the estrogen in the digestive tract and help remove it from the body. Try to get between 25 mg. and 30 mg. of food fiber per day. Some of my favorites include greens that are mineral-rich, too, like Swiss chard, spinach, broccoli, beet greens, mustard greens, sweet potatoes, kale, potatoes, green peas and green beans.

• **Add bioflavonoid-rich fruits** to help normalize body estrogen levels. Besides bioflavonoids, citrus fruits and berries are also rich in vitamin C, another nutrient that can help manage estrogen levels, decrease capillary fragility, facilitate the flow of nutrients and help remove the flow of wastes. Good sources of bioflavonoid foods are buckwheat, berries, citrus fruits (both pulp and pith) and grapes (including the skins). Vitamin C vegetables are another source of capillary strength to help reduce heavy menstrual bleeding often seen with fibroids (and endometriosis). Vegetables high in vitamin C include broccoli, cauliflower, kale, peppers, parsley, peas, tomatoes and potatoes.

*NOTE: For an ongoing healing and prevention diet, see page 22 ion the endometriosis healing section of this book. The key diet suggestions that boost the immune system against endometriosis also help to treat and prevent **fibroids**.*

B) Use herbs to alleviate breast tenderness, swelling and lumpiness, and normalize hormone secretions.

An effective herbal combination can be the "best friend" of women who are trying to overcome breast or uterine fibroids, ovarian tumors or prolapsed organs. Antibiotic properties help reduce inflammation and pain, allowing the body to begin to shrink the fibroid growths, elasticizing and toning tissue while it works. Phytoestrogen-containing herbs, especially, like dong quai (which also helps relax muscles and cramping), blue cohosh, licorice root and wild yam, act as estrogen and hormone balancers, reducing the effects of excess estrogen.

• An herbal formula, like Crystal Star's **WOMEN'S BEST FRIEND™** (with *goldenseal root, cramp bark, squaw vine, raspberry, dong quai, false unicorn, rose hips, sarsaparilla, peony and ginger* among others), helps reduce pain and inflammation, alleviates breast tenderness and lumpiness, and normalizes hormone secretions. It should be used for 3 to 6 months.

• Herbs also help balance a women's hormonal cycle by normalizing the liver, adrenal and pituitary functions. Six **EVENING PRIMROSE OIL** capsules daily or 2 TBS. flax seed oil help balance prostaglandin activity and provide essential EFAs; **MILK THISTLE SEED** extract supports better liver function.

• A plant-derived progesterone cream may be used locally on fibrous areas. Most successful formulas, like Crystal Star's **PRO-EST WOMAN'S DEFENSE™** roll-on gel contain whole wild yam (as well as *aloe vera, grape seed oil , fresh American ginseng, dong quai, damiana, licorice root, black cohosh, burdock root, sarsaparilla root and red raspberry* among others). Premier Labs also has an effective WILD YAM MOISTURIZING CREME, or apply a fresh comfrey leaf pack to nodules nightly.

⊷ Use herbs to reduce pain and inflammation.
Consider Crystal Star **ANTI-FLAM™** (with herbs like *white willow bark, St. John's wort, echinacea angustiforia root, white pine bark, gotu kola, red clover and devil's claw* among others) for soothing, as-needed help.

• Enzyme therapy from plant enzymes can help with both acute inflammation and infection. Consider PUREZYME caps by Transformation Enzyme Corporation.

• GRAPE SEED EXTRACT by NutriCology helps prevent the release and synthesis of compounds that promote inflammation.

• Add vitamin E, 400 to 800 IU daily, which helps normalize estrogen levels to help protect against excess estrogen effects. Vitamin E also has anti-inflammatory, hormone regulating effects.

C) An underactive thyroid is usually involved in fibroids. Iodine therapy from herbs and sea plants is effective. Two TBS. daily of dried, high quality sea greens, 2 caps, or 15 drops of sea plant extract, like Crystal Star **IODINE SOURCE™** extract, (with *kombu, kelp, dulse, alfalfa, spirulina, Irish moss* and other greens) can address all but the most severe iodine deficiencies.

• A hot seaweed bath with sea plants like those above can also be used for iodine therapy. The skin is the body's largest organ of ingestion. Iodine from sea vegetables is easily absorbed through the pores during a seaweed bath.

• Add snipped, dried sea greens, like dulse, kelp, nori, or wakame, to salads, soups, steamed vegetables or rice. Or use products such as: SEA SEASONINGS or dulse flakes by Maine Coast Sea Vegetables, or wakame or nori by Mendocino Sea Vegetables.

D) Love your liver. It's the key to long term estrogen balance.

Estrogen is secreted by the ovaries in a form called **estradiol**; the liver then converts the estradiol to an intermediary form called **estrone** and finally to a much safer, much less chemically active form called **estriol.** If the liver's function is impaired, this process is slowed down: the levels of the more harmful estradiol and estrone remain higher in the body and may stimulate breast and uterine tissue, worsening estrogen-dependent problems like fibroids.

One of the best ways I know of to help keep the liver healthy is to eat iodine-rich foods, chlorophyll-rich foods and liver and system-strengthening herbal supports like those found in Crystal Star SYSTEMS STRENGTH™ Drink Mix or capsules.

Key foods and herbs in this combination include *miso, soy protein, cranberry, brewer's yeast, vegetable acidophilus, alfalfa, oatstraw, dandelion, barley grass, licorice root, watercress, nettles, Siberian ginseng root, bilberries, schizandra, rosemary, dulse, wakame and kombu.*

Other recommended superfoods include: Nutricology PRO-GREENS, Green Foods GREEN MAGMA, Wakunaga KYO-GREEN, GREEN KAMUT by Green Kamut Corp., Transitions EASY GREENS , or VITALITY SUPERGREEN by Body Ecology.

Vitamin supplements can help your liver's performance, too.

• Include vitamin A; research shows that blood levels of vitamin A are significantly lower in women with excessive menstrual bleeding, a common symptom of fibroids. Almost 90 percent of the women in a recent study returned to normal menstrual bleeding after two weeks of extra vitamin A intake. I recommend beta-carotene or oceanic carotene, plant precursors to vitamin A, about 75,000IU. Good food sources of beta-carotene include sweet potatoes, carrots and romaine lettuce. One cup of carrot juice has 20,000IU of beta-carotene.

• Take vitamin C 3000mg daily with bioflavonoids to strengthen capillaries and minimize uterine bleeding. Bioflavonoids have estrogen-like effects to help balance the body's estrogen-progesterone ratio. **Vitamin C also promotes the absorption of iron.** (Note: if there is evidence of anemia, I recommend an herbal source of iron as an easily absorbed, non-constipating choice.)

• The liver also depends on an adequate supply of the B vitamins to metabolize fats and regulate estrogen levels. Good food sources of B Complex vitamins include lentils, pinto beans, black-eyed peas, black beans, lima beans, rice bran, corn, millet, barley and blackstrap molasses. Women with fibroids and related symptoms like excessive bleeding, endometriosis or premenstrual syndrome may also want to include a B-complex supplement.

Ovarian Cysts
You May Not Need Surgery For Ovarian Cysts

Ovarian cysts are becoming common today, especially in women with menstrual difficulties (either not having periods, or having excessive periods). Typical cysts are generally small, non-malignant chambered sacs filled with fluid. They are hormone-driven, usually stimulated by too much estrogen, and aggravated by specific unhealthy body conditions. But they are not cancerous, and are not thought to be cancer precursors.

Is surgery for removal of ovarian cysts your only choice?
The need for surgical removal arises not because of malignancy, but because the pedicle of the cyst becomes twisted and gangrenous, or because of painful pressure. They normally cease to grow after menopause, but they are often painful, especially during intercourse, and can cause excessive menstrual bleeding and inter-period spotting.

Although ovarian cysts are difficult to diagnose without a medical examination, there are some indicating signs:
1. acute or chronic pain in the fallopian tubes or ovaries
2. the inability to conceive a child
3. an erratic menstrual cycle with unfamiliar pain and unusual swelling and discomfort in the lower abdomen
4. painful intercourse, heel pain, and chronically swollen breasts
5. unusual abdominal gas, fever and coated tongue

Lifestyle elements that aggravate ovarian cyst development include current or previous use of an IUD, too much caffeine, a high fat diet, certain birth control pills, synthetic hormone replacement, and being overweight. Frequent radiation treatments and X-rays that you may undergo for other problems may change cell structure and set up an environment for ovarian cyst growth.

Diabetes, especially alcohol-induced diabetes, is a particular risky factor. A high-stress lifestyle encourages an over-acid system and therefore poor waste elimination, setting up unhealthy body chemistry for cysts.

According to the work of Dr. Catherine Kousimine, who has treated hormone-driven degenerative illnesses for over forty years, cysts and fibroids are formed when the liver isn't able to detoxify the body efficiently. She feels that cyst-type growths are created by the body as kind of a "second liver," as the body tries to deal with toxins and maintain its equilibrium. With this in mind, wholesome nourishment and the elimination of junk foods and other substances that contribute to the build up of toxins in the system becomes critical in avoiding cysts and fibroids.

Natural therapy for ovarian cysts focuses on normalizing hormone levels and correcting the unhealthy body imbalance that promotes cyst development. It gives your body a chance to heal itself, and offers you a choice before jumping into surgery.

In fact, I have seen the following therapy program work dramatically to help the body rid itself of abnormal growths like fibroids and cysts. In normal experience, it may take three full menstrual cycles for the typical growth to shrink in size or disappear. If the growths are dangerously large, you may wish to consider orthodox treatment or surgery, but get **at least** one second professional opinion.

Diet helps improve your body chemistry to overcome cysts.

Diet is an essential part of any natural healing program. It should be one of the first places to look as you develop a program against cysts. Once again, reducing your dietary fat intake is the first, best step to help lower estrogen levels and slow the growth of cysts. And, once again, saturated animal fats are the worst offenders. Avoid possible hormone-containing foods such as red meats, fatty dairy foods, eggs, and refined flour and sugars. Get the high quality protein you need for healing from whole grains, sprouts, soy foods, like tofu, tempeh and miso, fish, sea foods and free-range, "no hormone" chicken..

Emphasize a diet rich in dark green leafy vegetables, whole grains, legumes, nuts, seeds and fresh fruit.

Caffeine and refined sugars deplete the body of iodine, a nutrient you need for healthy thyroid activity and cyst protection.

Caffeine and sugars also promote over-acidity - an environment that encourages ovarian cyst development. Foods that are alkalizing and rich in B vitamins, like leafy greens and other fresh vegetables, miso, brown rice, wheat germ, brewer's yeast and sea vegetables are all good therapeutic choices.

Chlorinated water tends to leach vitamin E, a cyst protector, from the body. Try to drink only bottled water. Drink at least 48 ounces of water daily. Use herbal teas frequently.

Herbal therapy is effective against ovarian cysts and Type 2 PAP smears. Give yourself from 4 to 6 months of healing on an herbal, hormone-balancing regimen for ovarian cysts. The following program to reduce cysts has many years of success behind it.

• Take an herbal iodine source 2x daily like Crystal Star **IODINE SOURCE™** extract or **POTASSIUM/IODINE™** capsules. (See page 32 for formula). Or add snipped, dried sea greens, like dulse, kelp, nori, or wakame, to salads, soups, steamed vegetables or rice. Or use products such as: SEA SEASONINGS or dulse flakes by Maine Coast Sea Vegetables, or wakame or nori by Mendocino Sea Vegetables.

• Take 4 capsules daily of an herbal formula such as Crystal Star **WOMAN'S BEST FRIEND™**, (with *goldenseal, cramp bark, squaw vine, red raspberry, dong quai , false unicorn, sarsaparilla, rose hips, and peony*). In addition to its body balancing qualities, **WOMAN'S BEST FRIEND™** is anti-inflammatory to help reduce pain.

• Add four to six **EVENING PRIMROSE OIL** capsules daily.

• Add black cohosh extract to help dissolve polyp adhesions.

• Use dandelion or **MILK THISTLE SEED** extracts for proper estrogen metabolism through the liver.

• Enzyme therapy from PUREZYME caps by Transformation Enzyme Corporation, and GRAPE SEED EXTRACT by Nutricology also prevent the release and synthesis of compounds that promote inflammation and infection.

• **An herbal vaginal pack** can help draw out infection. Make it with powders of *echinacea root, goldenseal root, white oak bark, cranesbill and raspberry* with water and glycerine to make a solution. Use with a saturated tampon or a douche bag.

Continue your body balancing with a three month program:
Take two capsules daily of a **FEMALE HARMONY™** capsule combination from Crystal Star (with herbs like *dong quai, damiana, burdock root, sarsaparilla, oatstraw, nettles, dandelion, yellow dock , rosemary, peony, angelica and ashwagandha*) to help prevent return.

You may also wish to try the following nightly herbal douche to keep ovarian cysts from returning. It may be used 1 week on and one week off for a month at a time.

• In one quart of water boil the following herbs for ten minutes: one ounce each of raspberry leaves, black currant leaves, witch hazel leaves and powdered myrrh. Then simmer for half an hour and strain. Mix 4-oz. of the douche mix with a pint of boiling water; cool and use

If you have a Type II PAP smear, begin the following healing program:

✦ Effective herbal therapy:
• Crystal Star **WOMANS BEST FRIEND™** caps 6 daily, (see previous page for formula), or 6 goldenseal/echinacea/myrrh caps,
• Sun CHLORELLA, 1 drink, or 15 tablets daily,
• Six SHARK CARTILAGE capsules daily,
• Four PCO tablets daily, from grape seed oil or white pine,
• Four 500mg **EVENING PRIMROSE OIL** capsules daily.

Natural Therapies Offer Relief From Vaginal Yeast Infections

Vaginal yeast infections are becoming a scourge of modern times as women are more exposed to water and environmental pollutants, long courses of antibiotics, cortico-steroid and sulfa drugs, and frequent use of spermicidal preparations. In addition, poor diet, hormonal changes due to menopause or pregnancy, emotional stress, vaginal irritation from intercourse or excessive douching, birth control pills or hormone pills all contribute to yeast infections. For women that are prone to them, it seems almost anything can weaken immunity and change the chemistry of the vagina's delicate acid mantle, throwing body balance off. Yeast infections are, in many cases, a condition of pH imbalance rather than a disease.

The traditional drug treatment for vaginitis is antibiotics or sulfa drugs. Both are very effective in killing infection-causing bacteria but they also kill the good bacteria needed to maintain an ongoing healthy vaginal environment. In almost every case of orthodox drug therapy, the problems that created the vaginal imbalance in the first are not corrected, and the organisms begin to grow again. **In fact, the infecting organisms often multiply more quickly *after treatment* because the body's internal protective flora that once provided a natural defense have been destroyed by the antibiotics.**

A women seeing the infection return may take more medication, causing the cycle to repeat and augment itself again and again. The only way to treat yeast infections for permanent results is to correct the underlying causes.

Naturopathic therapy aims to re-establish normal vaginal flora, restore normal body pH levels and promote healing from within - in essence rejuvenate and balance the entire system.

Natural therapies are notably successful against vaginal yeast infections, but a long-term cure is not likely unless dietary and lifestyle changes are made.

A well balanced diet is critically important to clear a yeast infection. It also serves a woman well as a general preventive measure. **Sometimes a yeast infections can be cured by simply eating right.**

• Place your emphasis on whole food meals that center around whole grains, like brown rice, millet and buckwheat, fresh vegetables, especially leafy greens and steamed vegetables, like broccoli, cauliflower and peas. I recommend nourishing low fat soups, too, like miso, Oriental mushroom and vegetable broths.

• Include lots of lemons and grapefruit in the diet, but avoid eating oranges and other sweet fruits during healing. **Unsweetened cranberries and cranberry juice are highly recommended and help to restore acidity to the vagina.**

• Cultured foods should be included daily during your healing program. Foods like yogurt, cottage cheese, tofu, tempeh and raw sauerkraut are good examples.

• Avoid red meat and hormone-treated poultry during healing.

• Avoid all alcoholic beverages and all sweets during healing. Yeast feeds on sugar and alcohol. A yeast infection may be completely cleared just by eliminating sweets from the diet. If you have a raging yeast infection, it will be encouraged to grow by a diet that includes sugary foods.

Add plenty of probiotics. Friendly bacteria are critical to both healing and to protection against pathogens like yeast causing bacteria. They help replenish the flora normally found in a healthy vagina. Since dairy foods can sometimes aggravate yeast conditions, I usually recommend non-dairy acidophilus.

Here are some products we have tested that are effective probiotics:
• PROBIOTIC A. Y. (a yeast control formula for women) by Futurebiotics
• KYO-DOPHILUS by Wakunaga of America
• MULTI-DOPHILUS caps by Premier Labs
• DR. DOPHILUS by Professional Nutrition
• JARRO-DOPHILUS + FOS by Jarrow Formulas (Note: Fructo-Oligosaccharide (FOS) Is a microflora enhancer - a soluble fiber found in relatively high amounts in artichokes, onions, garlic, burdock, shallots, wheat, barley and bananas. It is difficult to achieve significantly high therapeutic amounts solely through the diet so FOS supplementation is often helpful.
• RAW SAUERKRAUT by Rejuvenative Foods
• ABC DOPHILUS POWDER by Solgar. (May also use as a douche.)

Here is a general anti-yeast tea you can use internally and as a douche.
Mix 4 to 6 tablespoons of herb mixture into a quart of water. Add cold water and bring to a simmer over low heat. Remove immediately and let steep twenty minutes. Strain. This is a bitter tea; you may wish to add cranberry juice for flavor.

2 parts sage	2 parts mullein
2 parts raspberry leaf	$1/4$ part goldenseal root

Vaginitis is a general term for the symptoms of vaginal infections from various bacteria, such as chlamydia, gonococci, strep and staph, or even from strong chemical douches or spermicides. Characterized by itching of the vulva area, sharp pain on urination, inflammation of the vaginal mucous membranes and external ulcers.

Natural therapies are generally effective.
• Take vitamin C crystals in water - up to 5000mg daily during healing, and use a weak water solution of vitamin C as a douche.
• An herbal suppository for chronic vaginitis might contain herbs like CRANESBILL, GOLDEN SEAL, ECHINACEA RT., WHITE OAK BK., and RASPBERRY. This formula can be made up at home by mixing the herbs with warmed cocoa butter to form finger-sized suppositories. Place the suppositories on waxed paper and put in the refrigerator to chill. Further specific use directions regarding making herbal suppositories can be found in HEALTHY HEALING Tenth Edition (page 446) by Linda Rector Page.

Leukorrhea is a typical multi-symptom yeast condition occurring when immune resistance is low or when normal vaginal acidity is disrupted. There is itching, irritation and inflammation of the vaginal tissues, foul odor, "cottage cheese" discharge, and painful sex. When the infection involves candida albicans yeasts, there is also lower back pain, itching and burning, chafing of the thighs, and frequent urination. Regular over-the-counter medication douches are ineffective for leuchorrhea.

Natural, especially herbal treatment, is often very effective for leukorrhea.
If the infection is mild, an herbal douche helps to rebalance the acidity of the vagina, rarely needing more than 3 to 4 days of application. An effective douche like Crystal Star's **WHITES OUT DOUCHE™** (with *witch hazel, squaw vine, comfrey, goldenseal, juniper, myrrh, white oak, pau d' arco and buchu*) may be used twice daily.
If the condition is more severe, add six capsules daily of an herbal combination with anti-biotic properties, like Crystal Star **WOMEN'S BEST FRIEND™** caps (See page 35 for formula.)

Two common types of yeast infections need extra treatment:
1) Trichomonas - a parasitic infection, found in both men and women; usually contracted through intercourse. "Trich" is characterized by severe itchiness and a thin, foamy, yellow discharge with a foul odor.

2) Gardnerella - a bacterial infection that thrives when vaginal pH is disturbed - also usually transmitted through sexual contact. Gardnerella is characterized by an especially foul, fishy odor, creamy white discharge, and moderate itchiness.

Here is an effective therapy program for trichomonas and gardnerella:
• Drink two glasses of sugar-free cranberry juice daily.
• Use a TEA TREE OIL vaginal suppository nightly for 2 weeks.
• Alternate salt water and vinegar douches every other day for a week.
• ake B and C complex vitamins to restore body balance.
• Use two strong herbal combinations that address a broad spectrum of infections. (Alternating the formulas every two hours keeps the herbs active in the body longer.)
    The first combination should have anti-biotic properties, like Crystal Star **WHITES OUT #1™** caps, (with *goldenseal root, myrrh, pau d' arco, echinacea, vegetable acidophilus, ginkgo and dandelion*).
    The alternating combination should have anti-fungal properties, like Crystal Star **WHITES OUT #2™** caps, (with *burdock root, juniper, squaw vine, bayberry, parsley root, dandelion, gentian, uva ursi and black walnut*).

- Take a good probiotic supplement (see probiotic products - previous page.)
- ANTI YEAST FORMULA by Jean's Greens (for treatment of yeast infections).
- PUREZYME by Transformation Enzyme Corp.
- DEFENZ by Premier Labs (anti-bacterial, anti-fungal, anti-viral product).

Vulvitis is an inflammation of the vulva, caused by an allergic reaction, irritation during sexual intercourse, bacterial or fungal infection. Characterized by itching, redness and swelling, it sometimes has fluid-filled blisters resembling genital herpes.

Effective natural therapies are very soothing. I have seen success with an aloe-based topical skin gel, like Crystal Star's **FUNGEX SKIN GEL™**, (with *pau d' arco bark, dandelion, gentian, myrrh, goldenseal root, witch hazel, and grapefruit seed*).

Other effective therapeutics include GREEN SALVE by Motherlove, HEAL ALL SKIN SALVE by Nature's Apothecary, and WISE WOMAN COMFREY COMFORT SALVE by Burt's Bees.

New Sexually Transmitted Diseases & Women

Sexually transmitted diseases are widely prevalent in our country today. It is estimated that one out of every five Americans has a sexually transmitted infection - among the highest in the industrialized world. The new ones are increasingly virulent, **and they affect women far more than men.** They can't be ignored. Reported cases only represent the tip of the iceberg. They are a significant health threat at every level of American life.

The more newly recognized STDs, such as chlamydia, venereal warts and cervical dysplasia are growing so fast they are being called new epidemics. There are four million new cases of chlamydia reported each year, the fastest rising STD in the country. Genital warts is also rising fast, particularly among women.

Most STD's are extremely contagious. Even though precautions may be taken during virulent stages when an STD is recognized, they can still be transmitted during inactive or quiescent stages. And because many people are asymptomatic after they are infected, an STD may be unknowingly spread for years.

Women are in greater danger then men.

Anatomically, women are more vulnerable to STD's than men, because a man's infected secretions remain in the woman's vagina after sexual ejaculation. If a woman has an STD, the man's exposure is short, because he ejaculates and withdraws. Women are also less likely than men to seek care, largely because most STD's have no symptoms in women, and current diagnostic tests are notoriously unreliable for women. Female-controlled prevention technology is not yet on a par with the male condom. Female condoms are still new and extraordinarily clumsy.

Sexual disease consequences are especially severe for women, because they are frequently irreversible and may be life threatening. They specifically damage the female reproductive area, often producing lingering infections, scarring and adhesions throughout the pelvic region which can prevent conception. The problem goes even beyond the woman herself. Her sexual responsibility may affect not only her ability to have a child, but through transmitted infection, her children's ability to have a child.

Here are the most severe complications for women from STD's:
- Infertility
- Potentially fatal tubal pregnancy
- Congenital infections passed to the newborn
- Low birth weight and/or premature birth
- HPV, (venereal warts), is a leading risk factor for cervical dysplasia and cervical cancer
- STD's increase the risk of HIV infection at least three-to five-fold

What are the best natural treatments for STD's?

For many years, the only treatment for sexually transmitted diseases was long courses of powerful, but immune-depressing drugs. Today, we are rediscovering the power of herbal remedies and other natural treatments against STD's. Some STD's respond better to natural treatments than others. Those with acute symptoms sometimes require a short initial course of anti-biotic drugs. But we are learning that a strong arsenal of herbal remedies and supplements can fortify the body against both outbreaks and some of the devastating consequences.

Ideally a doctor who is knowledgable about holistic methods can determine whether antibiotics or other drugs are necessary, or whether natural remedies alone will be effective. Even if conventional medicine is used, adding natural therapies under the supervision of a qualified professional with alternative knowledge can greatly assist healing.

It goes without saying that great care should be taken in selecting a safe sex partner, using latex barriers, and avoiding unsafe sex practices like anal and oral sex unless you have certain knowledge that your partner is free of disease. **It is of equal importance to optimize the body's natural immunity to infectious diseases. The immune system's strength determines risk for a viral disease, not just exposure to the virus or bacterium itself. Boosting the immune system with a good diet, supplements and herbs is a formula for success. For sexually transmitted diseases, it is important to maintain strong defense barriers in the digestive tract and skin.**

Doctors in many countries are calling Cervical Dysplasia the newest sexually transmitted epidemic. Cervical dysplasia is the formation of a precancerous lesion in the cervix. Researchers suspect that two sexually transmitted viruses, Human Papilloma Virus (HPV) and Herpes Simplex II are involved, because these viruses also play a role in cervical cancer. Since experts estimate between 40 and 80% of the young, sexually active U.S. population, is infected with either HPV or Herpes II, it is easy to see why cervical lesions are considered especially dangerous.

Can your lifestyle put you at risk for cervical dysplasia? Having multiple sex partners from an early age, smoking and a poor diet increase risk because it reduces immune defenses to create an environment for infection. Smokers are 3 times more at risk than non-smokers. Oral contraceptives are known to potentiate the adverse effects of nicotine, and to decrease the levels of key protective nutrients like vitamins C, B_6, B_{12}, folic acid, and zinc. Some oral contraceptives aggravate pre-cancerous lesions because of their imbalancing estrogens.

A woman in a sexual relationship with a man who has genital warts or herpes has an extremely high risk of developing a pre-cancerous condition of the cervix. Because the cervix is insensitive to pain, cervical herpes may infect without the woman's knowledge.

Here is a natural remedy program to help overcome cervical dysplasia lesions.

• A diet to encourage strong immune response against dysplasia is fiber-rich, low in fat and full of fresh fruits and vegetables. Particularly avoid sugary junk foods that aggravate herpes-type infections. Animal product consumption should be decreased, especially red meats and dairy foods because of their possible contamination with estrogens.

• Add anti-oxidants, especially the proanthocyanidins (OPC's from grapeseed or pine bark).

• There appears to be a strong relationship between low beta-caro-tene, low vitamin C, low selenium and B complex (especially folic acid and B_6) in the body, and the risk of cervical dysplasia. I recommend vitamin C, 5000mg, beta-carotene 100,000IU, and folic acid 800mcg daily.

• A protective herbal remedy with anti-viral activity against STD's would include herbs like ECHINACEA, GARLIC, LICORICE ROOT, DANDELION, WORMWOOD, KELP, PEPPERMINT OIL and L-LYSINE.

• Crystal Star **BIO-VI™** extract has both anti-biotic and anti-viral prop-erties. Or consider GOLD LABEL BOTANICAL USNEA & WELL-BEING LYSINE FORMULA by Zand Herbal Formulas, or FLOR*ESSENCE by Flora, Inc.

Note: Women with an advanced stage of cervical dysplasia may have a more natural choice for removing the dysplastic tissue. Some naturo-pathic physicians today use herbal "surgery," a process where the abnor-mal cells are "burned" off in a 3 to 5 week process with a twice-weekly application of zinc chloride solution and an herbal *sanguinaria* tincture. The treatments are accompanied by self-applied, nightly herbal and vita-min suppositories. For help in finding the nearest naturopath who per-forms this treatment (developed by Dr. Tori Hudson) call the American As-sociation of Naturopathic Physicians, 206-298-0125, to obtain a listing of qualified practitioners who use this approach.

Chlamydia is the most harmful of all STD's in terms of infertility for both men and women, striking an estimated 3 to 5 million people each year. It can afflict any part of the male or female reproductive tract, may be transmitted during either vaginal or anal sex, and regularly bounces back and forth between partners.

In women, chlamydia appears as a thick vaginal discharge. In addition to the vaginal/vulval area, it affects the fallopian tubes, endometrium and peritoneum. It may also infect the cervix, urethra, eyes, and throat. Chlamy-dia is responsible for over half of the 1 million cases of pelvic inflammatory disease, or PID, each year.

Chlamydia is most dangerous when there are no symptoms. If left untreated, it scars the fallopian tubes, causing total infertility or an ec-topic pregnancy, where the fertilized ovum implants in the tubes rather than the uterus. Always dangerous, an ectopic pregnancy may even im-peril the mother's life because it involves heavy bleeding, great pain, and life-threatening shock if there is a tubal rupture. Even if a successful uterine pregnancy is achieved, chlamydia increases the risk of miscarriage, prema-ture birth and instance of birth defects. An infant born with chlamydia it is at high risk for pneumonia, ear and eye infections.

Natural therapy for chlamydia increases circulation to the infected area, cleanses the blood, reduces inflammation and stimulates immunity.

Blood cleansing herbs have had the most success against chlamydia infection. Treatment should be started as soon as infection is known, and should continue for 1 to 3 months. Look for an herbal compound like Crystal Star **DETOX™** caps (with *goldenseal, red clover, licorice root, pau d'arco, echinacea, sarsaparilla, burdock, alfalfa, barberry, panax ginseng, garlic, kelp, milk thistle seed, and dandelion among others).* A new Japanese study found that berberine, an active constituent of such plants as goldenseal and barberry motivates macrophages, cellular scavengers that gobble up offending organisms like bacteria and viruses in the body.

The above herbal formula should be taken with:
• a daily green drink, and/or 15 Chlorella tabs daily,
• 6 garlic capsules ,
• 6 CoQ$_{10}$ 60mg capsules daily,
• beta-carotene 150,000IU and vitamin C, 5000mg. daily.
• Also consider INSURE HERBAL & THISTLE CLEANSE by Zand Herbal Formulas, and FLOR*ESSENCE by Flora, Inc.

Healing fluids with flushing and anti-inflammatory properties should be increased. I recommend cranberry juice, watermelon juice, carrot and cucumber juices to promote urination.

❧

Venereal Warts, or HPV (Human Papilloma Virus, are the most contagious STD, but the symptoms are often latent with an incubation period of three to four months. Almost 98% of infected individuals have no visible warts at all, even during the most contagious, early, pre-symptomatic period. So an infected person may spread HPV before he or she is even aware of it. Warts are most often passed during sexual intercourse with an infected partner, but can be picked up from objects that have been recently exposed to HPV and not properly cleaned, such as medical equipment or tanning salon beds.

Warts infect a woman's ovaries, Fallopian tubes, cervix, uterus and vagina. There may be painful, bloody sores in the genital area, or a chronic, heavy, pus-filled yeast infection, painful intercourse and high fever which can lead to brain damage.

HPV can be triggered by co-factors - like smoking, herpes, other STD's, and long courses of birth control pills. New studies show that HPV causes changes in the cervical cells and is now linked to cervical cancer. If you think you might have contracted veneral warts, an annual Pap smear is the most effective screening tool for detecting them. Natural therapy for genital warts takes about 6 months and is especially successful for women with pre-cancerous conditions of the cervix.

Herbal treatment for venereal warts focuses on a two-pronged attack - topical applications and oral anti-virals.

• Aloe vera gel along with 2 glasses of aloe vera juice daily is an effective topical application and anti-viral drink.

• An effective oral program includes two herbal compounds. The two compounds may be taken together, one week on and one week off until improvement is felt.

1) an extract like Crystal Star **ANTI-VI™** to overcome replication of the virus, (with herbs like *lomatium, St. John's wort, and bupleurum*).

2) a Crystal Star **FIRST AID™** heating formula to slightly raise virus-killing body temperature during acute stages, (with *bayberry, rosehips, ginger, white pine bark, white willow, capsicum*).

• an external topically applied **LYSINE/LICORICE GEL™** like the one from Crystal Star, (with *L-lysine, licorice root aloe and myrrh*).

• a *goldenseal/chaparral* vag pack mixed with vitamin A oil.

• Add folic acid 800mcg daily to help normalize abnormal cells,

• A daily supplement containing panax ginseng, germanium 150mg, vitamin C 3000mg, beta-carotene 150,000IU, and selenium 200mcg as anti-oxidants.

Many women are opting for safe, effective natural medicines. But, whether you choose conventional medicine, alternative healing avenues, or combine both in a complementary process, the real prescription for healing is knowledge. Most drug treatment offers short-term relief, but threatens long-term health. Educating yourself about natural medicines to deal with gynecological conditions gives you a choice.

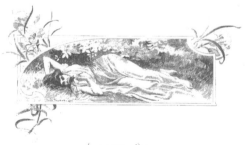